The Black Sheep

Striving to Live

Marie Sull

Table of Contents

Dedicated to "Rufus"

Your support for me and writing my story was invaluable

Thank you!!!

Introduction

The Black Sheep

Hello readers thank you for your interest in my book; I hope you enjoy reading my

story. You may even find that you relate to parts of my story, and I'm sorry about that.

If you read my story and you believe you may know me, please keep the information contained confidential. A few people in my life would not be comfortable with this book. I have decided it is time for me to share my story in hopes of helping others. Some things written in this book I have never shared with anyone, some things I have only begun to share.

Names, places, and dates have been changed in order to protect the innocent as well the guilty from any issues that could come from such a raw story. You may find I flip flop quite a bit from past to present and vice versa, however it has helped me too fully share my story with you.

Lastly, if you find your own story in what you read here please find someone you trust to confide in. If you do not have adequate support around you, please seek counseling from a trained professional. Don't give up, there is hope for you! You can recover and maybe one day I'll be reading the story of your life.

What are you supposed to do when truth is your enemy?

Foreword

How does one write a foreword to their life story? I guess I'll give it a try. I'm not even sure why I decided to write my story, but maybe someone needs to read it.

So let's get this boring part of the book over with, shall we? This book is true, it is my truth. It is about childhood abuse, rape, and the after effects. You won't find the real names or places associated with anyone in my story.

Sometimes I go into a Dissociative State or at least that is what my therapist calls it when I'm not exactly present or "with it". Disassociation is basically what the brain can do to avoid the pain of any given situation or memory. When you think about it, the disassociation really provides for protection. It protects the person from the trauma at the time, and later protects the person from the memories until they are ready to deal with them. Sometimes a current trauma can trigger a lapse and can cause a person to lose time or even get lost into a part. A part acts more or less like a protector or bodyguard over the person. It can be difficult at times to control disassociation episodes. For the most part outsiders do not see or even know about this condition.

It can usually be hidden quite easily. However, sometimes the person could have a breaking point, where his or her condition could come more to the surface, therefore bringing things to light. Sad to say this has happened to me. Let me tell you when it does you sure find out who your true friends are. I know that this is a hard condition to understand. I hope by sharing my story I can help more people understand.

Chapter 1

New Beginnings

I am curled up on the couch and staring at the computer page before me. Should I really call him? By this time I had looked at this page over a dozen times, as well as searched his name on the internet. He seems decent enough; he also looks warm and inviting. Can I really tell him my whole story though? Will he truly understand me or will he just repeat the same phrases I have heard for years?

The problem? He is a therapist... a therapist! Already the voices are going off in my head. "We don't trust therapists remember"? Why would he even listen to me, so I hung up the phone again for the 100th time. By this time I am wondering if his phone is showing my numerous calls.

"You are too much…" my former therapist's voice rings in my ears. He told me I was the reason he was leaving his practice and pursuing a different career. He said he had lost hope that I could ever get better. Imagine for a moment you are hearing this from your provider. Not only did he give up on me, he had lost all hope I would get better. Why am I trying again?

What if this Gary is just like Tim? I should note here that Tim really lost his practice because of some things he did to some of his other clients. He blamed me for losing his practice though, but what else is new? I was always blamed for everything bad that happened.

Just call me the <u>"Black Sheep"</u>.

My mind went back to when I first met Tim. Sigh…maybe this wasn't a good idea after all. Is it too late to cancel?

Calling Tim back and agreeing to counseling is a good idea right? I know him and I trust him I think. I have even talked to him, so what can taking this further step in my recovery hurt?

Is recovery possible for me after all these years? No one believes me and I'm the one left with all these memories and flashbacks. Remind me why I'm doing this again?

The morning of my first appointment with Tim and my stomach is acting like I am riding a rollercoaster. He comes out to meet me and I follow him slowly back into his office. I hate that the people in here know what I am here to see him for. I close my eyes as I sit down as if I am wishing I could snap my fingers and go back home.

13

Great, I have first time jitters and he is handing me paperwork. Do I really have to be here in this room? How did I get here? Why am I the one in therapy? Why am I the one that is crazy?

I was six; I thought it was the greatest thing to have a new daddy. Although, I longed for it just to be me and mommy in this house again. I was used to that. I don't remember my real daddy; he drowned and passed away when I was three.

I miss my real dad, although I still see his face and hear his voice. Would he be mad at me if I loved this new daddy? Would my new Daddy replace him?

My new daddy tells me I cannot go outside to play with my friends before dinner anymore. I whine to my mommy about it but she says I have to listen to him now, he's the boss. He has totally taken over the household as if he has been here with us from the beginning. Why did my real Dad have to leave?

Banished to my room again, Jenny and I play with my Barbies. No one knows but I talk to her when I am in my room or alone. She always says her tummy hurts and she doesn't like our new daddy. She was my only friend.

I pushed thoughts of Jenny away and try to focus on Tim's many questions. He is explaining how he wears two hats, one here and one at church. So basically he is saying he does not counsel clients in church. Blah… Blah… Blah… Oh yeah, I know him because we go to the same church.

Jenny would hate him because he is so serious and acts as if he has to tell me all his rules slowly. He must think I won't understand or follow what he is saying. I have been forced into therapy all my life and can probably recite the rules better than he can.

Why does he have to remind me that we are not friends? As if he would have even talked to me if it hadn't been for my family involving him in my life. I think his actual words were I am not in his "league". Great is my "crazy and untouchable" tattoo showing again? I hate that when that happens!

I don't really disagree with him, because if you had told me a few weeks ago I would be sitting across from him I would have said "Not on your life". I don't trust psych docs, therapists, or counselors. In fact, I even avoided him like the plague when I first visited the church where we attend. As soon as I found out he was a therapist, I wanted nothing to do with him. A lot of good that did me!

In my experience with therapists, all they want to do is label a person with some obscure sounding mental illness that makes you think that they know what they are talking about. Relax; I am not saying all therapists are that way, just in my experience.

If you are a minor just forget about it. Therapists will get you to trust them enough to tell them everything and then turn around and tell your parents everything you said. Again just my experience with a few jerks I was forced to see growing up.

I am so lost in my thoughts that I forgot where I was. I don't know if I really heard Tim the whole appointment. Oh well, it is time to go anyway. Yes!!

The light in my life greets me at the door, Blonde hair and blue eyes, just over a year old. I think I'll play with him a bit before I put him down for a nap. He always makes me smile! He loves our kitties, and always tries to take them to bed with him. First, we let our dog out and watch him run in the snow.

My son squeals at the sight of Buddy asking to come in. Bottle made, baby fed, baby in bed, check check check. Why is this day going so fast?

Now maybe I can clean before my husband comes home. Cleaning? Jenny would rather I draw with her. Shh!!!! No one knows she still exists and if anyone ever asks I'll just deny it. It is my plan anyway.

I sat down just for a moment and suddenly the realization hits me that I am back in therapy. That just plain sucks! Excuse the language but I never wanted to be in treatment again.

There is no doubt that I would not be alive if not for my baby. There is no way you can look at him and not think that he is the cutest baby in the whole world. I may be his mama, but my baby will be a heartbreaker when he grows up.

I looked at the clock and realize I have lost track of time and my baby is awake. I can't even tell you what I did those two hours, and I was sorry to see it end. Sorry to see it end but glad to see my baby again.

Snack time with baby and most of it lands on the floor. That is okay, because here Buddy comes to clean it up.

My husband walks in the door, and right off the bat I can tell he is in a bad mood. What else is new? Preparing for the worst, I put the baby in his playpen with some toys. No matter, he goes into the garage and slams the door as usual.

I found out my husband was mad again about his job and on the verge of quitting. So we start another fight which involves me begging him not to quit his job until he finds another job and him yelling about being told what to do. Sadly this happens often in our house. He has a problem with being told what to do in any situation, and

even jobs are no different. It does not help reminding him

of the baby's needs because he thinks we would save

money if I would just breastfeed. Never minding that I did

try, but it just did not work for me and baby. We go back

and forth before I give up and go and check on the baby.

Poor little one fell asleep on his toys; he reminds me that

this is worth it.

Why am I back in his office again? Did I really

agree to this? I don't even know where this week has gone.

I am again in this chair for another hour and a half

listening to his lame questions. I mean, why? Because after

all, thanks to my family talking to him Tim already knows

a lot about me and my situation anyway.

Something is making me feel uncomfortable with

Tim today. Yes, more uncomfortable than usual. I'm not

sure what it is, but something is different today. He

always acts like he knows me so well. Why? Just because we talked on the phone until he somehow convinced me to come see him for counseling? Why does he suddenly think he has all the answers about my life?

Tim is very intelligent, even charming to some people I guess. I hate that I am also charmed by him at times as well. In church, he is highly respected and I suspect a few church ladies even have a crush on him. Why am I here again? Please someone tell me why? I'm so tired of therapy and Tim, why can't I just go home?

I just know I can't tell Tim anything bad today, because it would make it awkward to see him at church tonight. I hate how he avoids me at church functions now like I am some disease to be feared, instead of a fellow church member. Not that he really paid all that much attention to me before I started counseling. It is just now he flat out goes out of his way to avoid me. It is actually funny watching him try to do this since he is the adult

Sunday school teacher, choir director, and a church Elder.

I wonder how Tim's wife feels sometimes,

especially when he works late at night. Oh yeah, did I say

how weird it is that her and I are friends?

Her name is Carol, she had beautiful hair and I

envied her then. After all she got to go home with Tim.

That had to be great right? Little did I know how unhappy

his profession made her at times. I once overheard her

talking to a lady at church about how clients contacted him

at all hours of the day. I vowed not to do that but some of

the things he brought up during sessions with him made it

difficult goal to accomplish. My friendship with her

though didn't last long. I soon learned that when he had

bad news to tell me he would wait until the end of a

session to break it to me. Sigh... today was one of those

days apparently.

I was gathering my stuff at the end of the session when he told me to hang on a minute. I slid into my chair and waited to hear what was up. He said "I know you like being friends with Carol, but I think we need to talk about it". "Okay, why?" I said. He went on to say that he didn't think it was a good idea for me to be friends with her because he felt I would get frustrated with her lack of time. You see Carol is busy and apparently as a crazy person I wouldn't understand that. Okay so that wasn't his exact words but they are pretty close. He said he felt like the friendship would cause me to "take a step back" in recovery. Take a step back; can I go any further back in his mind really? He reminded me again that I was not in their "circle". There's a Tim and Carol circle now? He didn't even care that tears were now falling down on my cheeks. "Now come on Ashley, you need therapy more than you need friends" he said. So this apparently was not really a "let's talk about this and come up with a solution", it was more of "this is how I decided it will be" talk. He didn't even act like he cared how I felt about it.

With that lecture he ended the long session. No, he didn't ask me how I was with that or will I be okay with this until next week? Decision made, talk given, case closed. I wasn't even allowed to say goodbye to Carol. According to him, it would not really be a big deal to her. I don't know what he said, but she never really approached me again.

Home again; I spent most of my baby's naptime crying. Trying to decide if it is really worth it and beneficial to go on seeing Tim for therapy anymore after today's little talk. If therapy hurts this much already, why am I willingly going through this again? Please say no! Please say no!

Thinking of my son, I had to give it a shot at least, even if Tim's rules did suck. Besides I did not want him to think he had won. It did hurt a lot but it was not like I haven't been through it before. Tim just pointed out the obvious that I was invisible and unimportant in this world.

I hate how the week goes so fast, and here I am again. Waiting for him to pull up outside, I thought about going out the exit before he saw me. I was lost in thought when he came out and called me in. Somehow he drew me in again, how did he always do that? What is wrong with me?

What an insult, he didn't even mention last week or his "little" talk he had with me. He is actually quiet for once and is staring at me. Oh I get it the therapist psych-out, the oldest game in the book. Doesn't he realize I know all this? I can be quiet and stare as long as he can. So I finally said "Look I am not talking today okay"? Yeah, I really thought that would fly.

He asked me why. I am thinking like duh you jerk. He said it is okay I'll wait for you to talk. That does not last long and lamer therapy questions that I won't bore you with. Only 30 minutes has gone by? Oh great a whole hour to go before I can leave.

My body starts hurting and suddenly I am back in my room. Jenny is showing me something. I am not ready for it yet and neither are you. I am suddenly aware of the tears on my face, great I'm still here? Ugh, his mouth is moving again.

-"Where did you go just now, Ashley hmm...?"

- "What do you mean?"

-"You were somewhere else and you were squirming".

-"No I wasn't I was right here".

-"Then what did I just ask you?"

- "You just asked me where I went just now".

- "Nope, try again. What did I ask you before that?"

- "Is this going to go on forever? Isn't it time for me to go"?

- "First tell me what I asked you".

- "I forgot okay? All your insane questions made me forget".

- "I want you write about this session, tell me what you remember about it".

- "Okay, can I go now?"

- "I want an answer, Ashley!"

- "Fine Tim, but for now I am leaving the room and that is my choice!"

Finally I am home, what a session. Why did he have to get so firm with me? Like I really knew where I was, and why didn't he? After all, I thought he knew all the answers. Besides that he asks me like he already knows the answer anyway, but what does he know? Why don't I know the answer or remember?

Oh no! What is my husband doing home? Great! This can't be good, and to top it off my mother is here. I walk inside and mom is sitting with my baby. I asked her when he came home, "Just after you left, and where did you go today again?" "Just a meeting mom, just watch the baby please while I go see what is going on with him."

"Nick why are you home so early"? I thought you worked today. "I quit". "What, I thought we agreed you would wait until you found another job!" "No, you agreed, besides you have a job so why are you worrying"? "It is not enough to cover our expenses and you know that"! "Well then, borrow some money from your mom to get us through". "Not again Nick, I'm tired of that and we need to take care of ourselves." "Suit yourself; now let me work on the car".

Great, another visit from mom that ended with me needing to ask for money again. Does she know how much I hate this scenario? No matter, she never hides her disappointment. I hear it in her voice and see it in her face.

I hid the money, hoping Nick wouldn't find it this time. Anytime he found it, he took it and spent it. If the money was going to pay enough of our bills, I needed to keep the money from him.

My life feels like a wreck; abuse I'm trying to get over, a deadbeat husband, and a 3 year old who hadn't started talking and was still in diapers.

In this stupid office again and Tim is staring at me again, doesn't he know how to do anything else?

-Well, Ashley do you have an answer for me?

- What question was that?

- Where were you if you don't know what I asked last week? Did you hear me?

- I spaced off okay? I guess I do that sometimes.

-Where do you go when you space off?

- I don't know okay?

- I think you do, so why don't you tell me?

- I don't want to talk about it.

- So, you do know, you just don't want to answer me.

- You got it Sherlock, time to go bye-bye!

- We'll discuss this next time.

-Whatever.

Chapter 2

Answers?

So probably by now you are wondering, whatever happened to Gary right? There will be plenty of time for that later. If you want to understand what happened, I need to give you some background information.

Two weeks without therapy is a long time even if you are not sure you like it. He was transitioning to his new office. Just when I was feeling safe, he goes and changes his office location. A lot can happen in two weeks you know right? Already I hate this new place, too many people and it's hard to get way out here.

He is ready for me to come back, but I don't think I am ready for a session with him today. "Well Ashley..." he starts out, I think I may have some answers to what has been going on with you".

- Do you know that you signed your journal different this week?

- What do you mean? So what?

- You signed your journal "Jenny" and even your handwriting is different.

- So? Sometimes my handwriting is different, big deal.

- It is a big deal, and I'm going to tell you why.

Why is he looking like a kid on Christmas morning? His grin is sickening. He is even getting closer to my chair and I don't like that at all.

"Ashley, I believe you have Dissociative Identity Disorder, do you know what that is"?

You mean Multiple Personality Disorder? Well yes, but isn't that rare?

Yes, but the spacing off, nightmares, and losing time are all telling me this is a real possibility with you.

So I'm crazy now?

No I am not saying that but learning about it may help us to understand what is going on so we can deal with it.

"I don't want to learn about this, the idea is crazy".

With that I started crying, and you will soon see that I hate even the thought of crying in front of someone else. He handed me a Kleenex and I snatched it like I might be afraid he'll take it back. Great there is almost 45 minutes left of the session.

- Are there any others?

- What do you mean?

- Are there others besides Jenny?

- No!!!

- I think there is Ashley.

- Stop okay? I need time to process all of this!

- Do you want to get better?

- I thought you said I wasn't sick.

- You aren't sick but you need to deal with this.

- Why? So I can keep paying you?

He laughed and said no so you can feel better. "How old is Jenny?"

-"I don't know"

- Yes you do, Ashley.

- If you know, why don't you tell me?

- Because I don't want this!

- Now that we know this is what is going on, let's deal with it.

- Do I have a choice?

- You always have a choice.

-It doesn't feel like it.

- I think we should discuss increasing sessions to twice a week.

- Next time.

Twice a week though? It is hard enough for me to get a babysitter once a week, let alone get there! It did not really feel like I had a choice. Sigh.. I'll probably try. After all, I'm not ready to accept this diagnosis.

You don't really need to hear all this do you? Just a lot of arguing and therapy talk, nothing new. I'm not a brat, I'm usually nice but he is starting to make me angry here. Why is he so sure I have this thing? This MPD/DID. So with that, he ends the session by telling me to write about Jenny and write if there is any other "parts" inside me. All I was concerned with at that point was leaving and getting the heck out of there. He called me at home later that night to see if I was okay. I didn't even call him.

Okay? Sure yeah you just diagnosed me with a serious mental illness that you say will most likely require lifelong therapy but sure I am okay. Who did he think he was?

Chapter 3

Someone new

Do you mind if I take a break? We could even talk about Gary for awhile. Don't worry there is also a Rufus, no that is not his real name but he chose Rufus for his name when I started this book. He's a real comedian he makes me laugh, but he did something Gary and Tim combined could not do. More about "Rufus" later, I am sorry I have lost track again. That happens a lot; probably why he thinks it is DID huh?

I'm standing out in the hallway; Gary is not even here yet. Why did I make this decision? Well we have talked several times since I called him the first time. Midwest + bad weather= Rescheduled appointments. Is it too late to leave?

There is a guy coming this direction in what looks like a thick leather jacket. He kind of chuckles and says

"You must be Ashley; I'm Gary I will be with you in a moment." Of course he hands me paperwork to fill out, yuck. I'm so jumpy I barely notice him come out to usher me into his office.

"So what brings you here, Ashley?" Oh barf, didn't we talk about this enough on the phone? I'm quiet for awhile. "Yoo-hoo are you with me?"

- Sorry it's just… I trailed off.

- It's just what?

- I didn't want to be here again.

- Be where?

- Why? By now he is staring intently at me.

- It's a really long story.

- Well, we have an hour and a half. But let's go over the rules and general information first okay?

- Okay I sighed and settled in to listen to what I already know.

- He must have seen my look of disinterest.

- Why is this a sore spot with you Ashley?

- Been there, done that, bought the T-shirt.

- Alright, Alright but let's go over some basics.

Why am I here again? I don't want to be, I don't want to be. Whoops, he's mouth is moving again I guess I better pay attention. I do not want Gary to worry or even know about my so called diagnosis. Oh oh I think he noticed I trailed off again. Great!

- Where were you just now?

- What do you mean?

- Come on, do not play this game with me!

- I guess I just was not paying attention.

- Did this ever happen with Tim?

- If you want me to be honest, we probably shouldn't talk about him yet.

- Okay, well let's end for today and pick this up next time.

- Okay, thank you.

- But I want you to think about what you want out of therapy.

- Why do therapists always ask that?

- Because it is what we do, see you Thursday.

I am not really sure I want to go through all this again with therapy. No offense to Gary he does seem nice, but I am so done with this process. I'm so sure about this apparently, that I called him to leave him a voicemail. I nervously said that I was not sure I wanted to continue therapy and could he give me a call back before Thursday. To my dismay, he called back 20 minutes later. He said he had a few minutes and wanted to return my call. Of course he asked why I wasn't sure about continuing therapy with him. I said because I have been in some kind of counseling most of my life and what happened with Tim really made me distrust therapists. He said he wasn't Tim and would like me to come in Thursday to discuss the issue further in person. I reluctantly agreed but I was already thinking of not showing up Thursday.

Thursday came and because of my ride I got there 30 minutes early for my appointment. Since he had a small office I decided to wait downstairs instead until my appointment. I'm sitting on a bench reading for about 15 minutes and someone comes over and says "Hello". I look up and it is him! He said I'll see you upstairs as he enters the elevator. I toy with the idea of leaving without seeing him. In the end I decide that it wouldn't be nice if I just didn't show up. Sigh… I trudge up the stairs and he ushers me in.

- I'm glad you decided to come in today.

- I almost left at the last minute.

- Why?

- I told you, been here done that and bought the t-shirt.

- So why did you contact me then?

- Things were coming up again in my life.

- Like what?

- Stuff that…

- I'm not sure I can talk about.

- You came in today.

- Because you told me too.

- You know it was your decision.

- That doesn't mean I'm ready to talk to you.

- You can say whatever you need to in here.

- Isn't it time to go?

- No, we can stay here and talk awhile.

- This is scary.

- I know

- No you don't, you are on the other side of all

  this.

- Why are you here?

- You already know.

- Let's talk about it.

- Fine, whatever.

- So, why are you seeking therapy again?

I won't bore you with the rest of that second session.
Truth I was really nervous and I really didn't know if it
would be possible for me to continue seeing him anyway.
He sensed the nervousness and we talked about it. Finally
it is time to go and we set up an appointment as well as a
time to talk it over on the phone.

Home again; I'm still questioning this whole therapy
thing. However; since I'm in the whole process of deciding

whether or not to report Tim maybe it would help to talk it through in therapy.

- You're back

- Yeah, yeah take a picture it will last longer.

- Have you decided to continue therapy with me?

- I don't know…

- Can I help you decide?

- I don't know…

- That's not an answer.

- Well I don't know yet okay?

- What is holding you up?

- I hate therapy.

- Understood, why?

- I have basically been in and out of therapy since I was little.

- Why?

- Parents, school, and after court…

- Oh? After turning your stepdad in?

- My friend turned him in.

- Same difference.

- Whatever.

- You like to argue don't you?

- I don't know, I guess.

Same old therapy stuff, different office, different day. Will I go back to Gary? Probably; he does seem okay but please don't tell him I said that.

Chapter 4

Him Again?

I wonder if Tim knew I'd write about him someday. He probably wouldn't have thought I would since he seems to have been surprised that I was not locked up somewhere. Sigh… back in Tim's office again. Why am I here again? Right away he starts with the questions.

- Did you bring your list?

- You know I still think that I don't have this DID crap.

- Why don't you let me be the judge of that?

Ugh… he is getting closer again. Hasn't he ever heard of personal space? He is just staring at me while he reads my "homework". He is getting so close my only defense is to draw up my knees. Just because I know him does not mean I trust him in that way. He needs to back up now. He says he just wants to see my face, well then back up you creep. For a so called bright guy he sure does not pick up signals very well. I guess I don't really appreciate when anyone gets too close but he is crossing the line. I feel like I can't tell him though, so I just draw my knees up tighter. I can't wait to get out of here. He is staring at me again, but he hasn't backed up yet. I guess this is a smaller office but still, space please.

- Did you list all the parts?

- Yes, but I told you I don't think this is real.

- I think it would be helpful if we talk about this.

- Whatever.

- We still have time left; do you want to talk about this?

- Do I have a choice?

- You always have a choice; I actually had a cancellation if you want to stay longer.

- Okay I'll stay.

- But that means we need to talk.

- Whatever

Looking back, I argued with Tim quite a bit. I didn't trust him and I was starting to see why I should have never seen him.

His mouth is moving again. Not sure if I am really listening, he is telling me about Dissociative Identity Disorder. I can't believe I am still sitting here, where is the door?

Did I mention I am engaged to my second husband? Tim doesn't like him; I found that out when I told him. He almost seemed jealous of him. His response was that he didn't think I would concentrate on therapy if I was getting married. He was wrong because my soon to be husband was very supportive. Well he was at first, and then he decided he didn't like Tim. I should have listened to him.

Therapy with Tim soon took over my life and it ruined my marriage.

Tim only decided he liked John after we got married and I used his insurance to pay for therapy. He still charged me personally though. This really means he was double billing because his whole fee was covered but I didn't realize it. My husband wanted me to stop seeing him, but I needed therapy. Problems with home life and past abuse were taking over my life.

I didn't like therapy but I thought it would help me with my life, marriage, and my son. I wanted a better life and didn't realize that therapy was slowly making it worse. By that time I had been in therapy with Tim for about 3 years. I thought Tim was helping me but I didn't realize he was really just grooming me.

Funny, since grooming was a term I learned from him. He said that it was Burt who really groomed me.

Gaining my unwavering trust so I would do whatever he asked me to do. Tim was right, I knew better than to go against Burt.

I tried telling him about what happened with Burt as me, Ashley. But he called out Jenny and other little parts as often as he could, insisting that I let "them" talk. Sigh.. it would be difficult to tell him about Burt.

Chapter 5

Step Monster

I guess I should talk about what brought me to therapy in the first place. I really should say stepdad instead of "step monster" but he does not really deserve that title either. He will also never replace my dad, even if my mom has replaced him in her heart.

Burt took over our lives and the household before they were even married. Early in their relationship I accidentally spilt pop on his favorite record and ruined it. I was 6 but he decided he would never forgive me for that mistake. He was also mad at mom for not punishing me for the accident. Burt didn't allow for mistakes and you best not point out his mistakes. At first I thought it would be great to have a new dad, but I soon found out Burt was someone to be feared.

He would get mad over everything. My mother was overprotective before he moved in but at least she let me do things. I played outside after school; I went to friend's houses to play and for dinner. Burt thought that was inappropriate so I was no longer allowed to play outside and join my friends. Burt wanted to know where I was at all times. Soon after that he even stopped me from going out to play after dinner.

I was born with Cerebral Palsy due to complications during delivery. It only affected my left side, so mostly my mother just allowed me to play for physical exercise. Burt stopped that to because he felt my mother was going too easy on me. Soon I was working out every night, while my friends played outside.

I had a favorite night gown that I wore when I was little; it was light blue with a ruffle at the bottom and had characters on it. I held to it even when it was getting shorter and shorter on me. I don't remember when he started to come into my room at night, but Jenny was right something was wrong with this new daddy.

I slept with a blanket and the same stuffed animal every night; they were from my birth dad and no one was going to take them away from me. Burt and my mom tried several times to remove the blanket; I even fished them out of the garbage.

I started to get urinary tract and bladder infections all the time. My mother and doctor thought the infections were caused by poor hygiene, they had no idea what was really going on at night. Much to my embarrassment my mother started to help me clean my privates. It didn't help that I often wet the bed at night, I slept deep but I was also terrified to get out of bed. There was no such thing as bathroom privacy anymore. Even Burt was taking an unwelcome interest in my bathroom habits. This occurred well into my teen years and still confuses me today.

Burt was paranoid, always worried about what would happen and he usually came up with the worst case scenarios. Before long I had passwords I needed to remember when I was picked up from school. If the person did not have the correct password I was not to go with them, no matter who they were. I know this is a normal occurrence with families, but Burt would test me and I would get in trouble if I didn't respond the correct way. He also constantly changed the passwords, so it was hard to remember them. When I was finally allowed to stay at home by myself, I was only allowed to answer the phone if it rang a specific amount of times. He would choose different patterns and I better not get those patterns wrong either when he called. When I was 14 he taught me how to use a handgun, and I was instructed to shoot would be intruders and one specific family member if he should come onto our property. He told me I trusted people too much, and most people could not be trusted.

I started to zone out in school and started falling asleep in physical therapy. My school day and afternoons were full of professionals looking after me; maybe I should have told them what was going on. After all they kept asking why I zoned out and kept falling asleep. I was scared though, and my mom and Burt put on a good show in front of people. I did not know who they were trying to fool, but people bought it. They had professionals believing I was the problem because I had behavioral issues. I wasn't a bad kid; I just couldn't pay attention and had taken to harming myself.

My mother was as much of a victim as I was, Burt controlled her every move. If she brought something for herself that he didn't like she had to return it to the store.

She was required to call him whenever she got to where she was going. I can see how someone might want to do that when traveling a long distance, but this was even for short trips. I couldn't turn to her for comfort because Burt was abusing her also just not in the same way, or was he I wondered?

When I was old enough, I do remember wondering what was going on behind closed doors at night. I mean why did he always have to come to me, and why didn't she know that he was coming to me?

I mean Moms should know these things shouldn't they? Did we really hide it that well? Didn't she wonder why I didn't like being alone with him? Why there were stains where there shouldn't be stains? She always found reasons because she couldn't bear to think that Burt was any less than perfect. To this day she still insists Burt was a good father to me. What is her definition of a good father?

There were the constant infections and behaviors that would have suggested possible sexual abuse. I remember people asking me but my mom and Burt were usually in the room with me. How exactly was I supposed to say anything? I am not sure I even was old enough to understand and realize what was happening anyway and just how wrong it was. I know what you are thinking, but it became my normal. I prepared myself for him to come into my room. It seemed the best way to just get it over with. After all, It was going to happen anyway right?

So what was the point of telling people who did not listen to me anyway? My saddest memory of trying to tell someone was in High school not long before Burt was actually turned into the police. A student teacher, let's just call him Joseph, began tutoring me in the class because I was struggling with the class.

I never really struggled with classes until that year and I would often fall asleep in school. He started asking me questions about my home life and slowly I opened up to him, except the deep stuff and he never asked leading questions. At some point I did share enough that he shared his concerns with the main office. He was not there the next day or the next. I learned that between Burt and the main office his assignment at my school was terminated. I was devastated and lost, the one person that I had trusted was gone and to this day I have not been able to locate him to thank him for standing up for me. He gave me to the courage to tell my story when I finally did break away. I only wish I would have had the courage to let him in a little more.

I turned into the good girl again, but I knew after that happened I had to find a way out. I ran away a total of two times and Burt was turned in the second time. Burt always found out where I was, looking back I'm sure he threatened my friends and their parents. He threatened one parent with a charge of kidnapping, even though I was there of my own free will. After playing the part of being angry, he tried making promises to me that I knew were a lie. I know I skipped many years ahead here, but I'll get there.

That second time I ran away was the last time I saw Burt, but in some ways he'll always be with me. I knew he'd always find me, threatening to hurt those who helped in any way. It wasn't enough that he took away my innocence, he was determined to keep a hold on me whatever the cost. He cost me my friends and my mom.

The real cost was actually much higher than I ever imagined.

Chapter 6

My Mommy

I woke up from my nightmare to find myself in an office; Tim is staring at me again. "Ashley, where did you go?"

"Nowhere, I am right here"

- You know what I mean.

- Nope. Why don't you tell me what you meant?

- Do not play games with me Ashley, it won't help.

- So I was zoned out so what?

- Do you know where you went?

- Just remembering that last day.

- What about that last day?

- Hearing Mom crying and wanting to run to her.

- You told me you had an attitude with the police.

- I'm not talking about that, besides I was scared to death.

- Why didn't you go to your mom?

- Burt was there, and besides two policemen were with me in the room.

- Didn't you care about what she was feeling that night?

- What about me? What about what I felt that night?

- You weren't a little girl anymore.

- Yes I was, I was Jenny curled up in the chair. I was terrified.

- Do you want to rock in the chair today?

- No. I just want to sit.

- I can help you feel better.

- No you can't, no one can. It won't ever be better.

- It won't get better if you don't try.

- Can I just go now?

I'm not sure if I waited for his answer or I just got up and gathered my things and unlocked the door. Yep, he locked the door.

Forgive me my timing is so confusing with my therapy with Tim. In actuality I remember only a handful of sessions, though I was in therapy with him for several years. Imagine years of appointments running together, it didn't even feel like several years of therapy. It took me awhile to realize just why it did not "feel" like actual therapy. It took taking a total break from him to realize it. No follow up and no contact from Tim, it finally meant I was alone with my thoughts. No more "parts" to protect me from the flood of emotions.

So, did I care about how my mom felt that night? Sure. But no matter how old I was that night, I needed my mom. Where was she? She was by Burt's side. I never was really told the truth about whether or not he was arrested, though he often whined about being in lock up.

My mom sure didn't care how I felt that night inside a locked group home. It took her over a week to come see me and it wasn't a pleasant visit. I get it, she was scared of Burt but I was her daughter.

What is strange is the conflict I felt those first few nights at a place when my every move was watched. I wanted my mother but yet I did not want to be near her at all. After all where had she been? I was her little girl before Burt was her husband, yet she believed him and not me.

She lied; she lied to the police and the counselors, said I was never alone with him. Burt worked days, while mom's schedule often varied. In earlier years, I spent mornings and afternoons with a sitter until her or Burt got off work. But in the later years when I was finally allowed to go home after school instead of a sitter, sometimes Burt got home first.

Sometimes when he was off from work, I'd already find him in my room afterschool. So how can she say I was never alone with him? More still why would she be afraid to leave me alone with him? This is a man she married after all; shouldn't she be okay with him being around her daughter?

It wasn't all her fault, as I said earlier she was his victim too. It was obvious I couldn't tell her anything, when she was afraid to breathe wrong around him. When I was younger I had thought my mom was so strong, but Burt, Burt turned her into a weak person.

Our relationship presently is anything but normal, for years after Burt was turned in, it was nearly nonexistent. She blamed me for splitting up the family. She tried to hold the court records against me numerous times, years later I found out just what she didn't want me to see them. Was the decision totally favorable towards me? No. But the decision was not totally favorable towards her and Burt either. I was taken from their custody by the State. Sure it meant two group homes and an uncertain future, but I was free.

After a few weeks in a home outside the city, I was moved back to one in the same city my mom worked in. I was happy; I was helping to cook lunch and consoling a new friend who was told she was going to be sent back home. My mother came to visit and asked if I wanted to move in with my grandparents. This from someone who had gone along with Burt and wanted me to be locked away somewhere. I did not have time to adjust; it really was not a question. I was thrilled but also scared. It would mean I was still under my family's thumb, and a new school for my senior year. No chance to even say goodbye to the few friends I did have. Sometimes I wonder where I would be if I had refused, all I knew is what was threatened. So I put my few belongings back into a garbage bag and left with my mom the next morning.

Though my mom tried, there were still many fights and times where things fell apart. Shortly after I moved in with my Grandparents, she called begging me to say that I had lied. I heard Burt yelling in the background. She pleaded as I asked what was going on there. Burt was threatening to leave. She called so many times that night; my Grandma took the phone cord from the wall. She reminded me that though I was her granddaughter, my mother was her daughter. What was I supposed to do with that?

I wanted to crawl into a hole, because I understood what she meant. However I also understood that I was the kid in this situation. Why couldn't mom protect herself? What did Burt have over her anyway? Why didn't she just say she knew what he did to me? Why didn't she kick him out of the house? Why did she ship me off?

At times, I went back and forth whether I should lie and say it never happened, so I could protect my mom from Burt's wrath. Sometimes all I wanted to do was run back into my mother's arms. What would that do though? Would me going home really "save" her? What would going home do to me? I was told so many times to think about what this is doing to my mother, don't you love her? No one ever said "I'm sorry; this must be hard on you". So yes, I was torn between going back to uncertainty and staying where safety was assured. Did I love my mom? Is that even a valid question? Of course I did! However sometimes even the people we love are not safe to be around. Years later, I still sometimes long for what will never happen. Yuck, there's that longing word again.

Chapter 7

Dead Inside

I soon settled into life at my Grandparents and soon school was out for the summer. It seemed odd not to panic at the thought of being home all day. But soon I was forced into counseling again.

Something started to happen inside of me, I'm not even sure what or how to explain it. I tried to be good for my Grandparents and concentrate in school but something raged inside of me. Rage was a dangerous feeling for me.

I started leaving the house for long walks, sometimes even overnight. My Grandma often worked nights, so it was easy for me to leave the house unnoticed. I didn't do anything but in a small town I could walk miles and miles. Nightmares often kept me awake and I needed the distraction. I soon was able to stop myself from feeling anything, or at least I thought. I started to become dead inside. I became dead to my feelings, dead to my longings, and dead to love. That is possible right?

Strangely enough, shutting off my feelings brought new life to me. I was able to concentrate in school and started cooking for my Grandparents. It gave me some sense of purpose to cook for my Grandpa when my Grandma was sleeping off the night shift. My Grandma allowed me to do things around the house that I was never allowed to do at home. I was finally home and had what I had so desperately wanted, or so I thought.

Wanted? Longings? Yikes isn't this chapter called "Dead Inside"? Well it went back and forth, well anyway anyone who says they are dead inside is lying.

Humans feel and humans long, it's in our nature. However I still tried to avoid any sort of longing. I still tried to live as if I didn't feel or want anything. Who wants to feel? I told you feeling is dangerous.

I'm not sure if I actually succeeded or if I was fooling myself. Now I know I was fooling myself then but I was only a teenager. But then, it seemed to make things easier for me. Feelings were dangerous and longing for something, anything was disastrous.

My grandparents tried to make their house a home for me. I never did without and I was allowed privacy. Privacy? I'm not sure I knew the meaning of the word but I loved it. My Grandpa was much respected in the church and at times that made it very hard to be his granddaughter. I was once taunted and repeatedly slapped for being a "goody two shoes". I never told them and soon the marks went away. I was terrified of being taken from them. Already several of my family members were trying to convince my Grandma that she and Grandpa could not possibly take care of me, that I would take advantage of them. Yep, there's my black sheep tattoo showing again. I have never seen it but it must be there.

My only struggle in obeying my Grandma was over the phone, long distance calls cost money. My few friends lived out of town. But soon enough I settled down and stopped the calls, disappointing Grandma was not an option in my mind. Mind you, these were the days before cell phones and Face book was an option, imagine that.

Where was I? Oh right right dead inside. I did not want to feel anything and no matter what it took I was determined not to feel. Soon I resumed ways to push feelings down, I self harmed for years at home so I just picked it up again. At first it hurt, but soon I was once again able to push away the pain. A roommate of mine at one of the group homes self harmed quite a bit when she

could get away with, but like I said we were watched day

and night. I didn't care what I was doing to myself; I just

did not want to feel anything. When you are abused,

feelings seem dangerous. They leave you feeling

vulnerable and helpless.

Being vulnerable and helpless was not a good way

to be! Okay, so I still feel that way at times. Okay a lot of

times, but I am trying to look at it differently. That is

possible right?

Sometimes I stockpiled different kinds of pills and

took them. Not enough to kill myself, but enough to zone

out. Relax nothing illegal, over the counter stuff. However,

one time I did take enough to scare me, so I made myself

throw them up and didn't tell anyone. At that time I didn't

think anyone would have cared if I had died. Besides

especially at that moment I was the "Black Sheep". My so called family had all but used those exact words. I know they saw me as a burden. Feeling like a burden on everyone made me want to escape even if it meant I was escaping my Grandparent's safety. But why would you want to escape safety you ask? Because I didn't know how to handle safety, it was not normal for me. Chaos, now that was normal for me. After all wasn't everyone's life like that? Wasn't chaos normal? Wasn't abuse normal?

Safety was not normal for me, if anything I was suspicious of it. When my Grandpa would come in and wake me up in the morning, I would freak out. I was still afraid of a male entering my room. I would try to take baths when he was napping because I was afraid he would walk in on me. Yes, it still happened as I'm sure it happens in other households. But I didn't trust males.

Oddly enough I had a different experience when it came to school in that new town. Quite the opposite actually, I respected the male teachers while I did not trust the female teachers. I'm not sure whether it was the last trimester of the school year or the first trimester of the next school year but everything was going fine until one questionnaire changed everything.

Chapter 8

Teachers

Small town schools are different; there is no hiding in the back of the classroom. One teacher in particular paid extra attention to me, and it went downhill from there.

Funny thing is years later he wound up taking the position of principal; I shuddered at that thought though I was never in trouble with the principal. Although he did once wince at what I was wearing, but never said a word. Then again, thinking about what I wore that day I wince.

Mr. Anderson taught business and math courses. That first day I was nervous anyway, he was so cute! Give me a break I was a teenager! Worse these subjects were not my best school subjects. He handed out a "get to know you" questionnaire. The sight of it made me sweat bullets. The question "tell me about yourself" danced in front of me. It was our first assignment for the class. I didn't complete it, and I always did my homework. I mean what was I supposed to say?

My mother had already made me lie to the principal and school counselor about the reason I had moved there. It made me sick how easily the lie had rolled of her lips. So what do I write the lie? It just didn't seem right.

I managed to sit through a class and two class periods out in the hall without completing what most would think was a simple assignment. I wrote like two sentences and handed it to him. He said it wasn't enough and I had to stay after school to finish it. I told him I didn't know what to say. When he came out of his classroom I hadn't written anything yet and he ushered me in to sit down. He asked why this was so tough for me.

Something he said made my tough shell break, and I blurted out the whole thing in tears. I think it took him forever to blink or move. I cannot even remember what he said before he let me go, but he made me promise to see him before classes the next day. I promised but begged him not to call my Grandparents.

I cried the whole walk home from school. What did I do? I was already threatened by then what would happen if I told the school the real story. What would he think? Worse what would he do? Would he tell the principal and the school shrink? As I walked in the house I wiped my tears away so Grandpa wouldn't see and washed up to make dinner.

When I woke up the next morning, I was hoping I dreamed the whole thing. Nope no luck, Mr. Anderson was waiting for me in the hallway. Unlucky for me, I had free time before my first class. He was starting to remind me of Joseph.

He had me take a seat and closed the classroom door. I think I saw tears in his eyes as he sat down. Suddenly I am sorry I did that to another teacher. I honestly didn't mean to, I tried. Stupid assignment.

He asked me how I was and if I remembered what I told him. Let's see; couldn't eat, couldn't sleep, yep I remembered.

- Mr. Anderson, I don't know why I told you all of that. Can we just forget about it please?

- Ashley, I cannot forget what you told me.

- Please Mr. Anderson I'll get in trouble.

- From who?

- From my mom, from the principal, from my Grandparents.

- I think it's your Grandparents that should be worried, and why are you worried about the principal?

- Wait why my Grandparents?

- Ashley, it's time for class, come talk to me during lunch.

- But why my Grandparents? Don't please!

- Ashley, you'll be late, come to my classroom during lunch.

I couldn't concentrate in classes, and almost got in trouble for not paying attention. Another school, another day more teasing as I make my way back to Mr. Anderson's classroom. Why does this seem like I have done this before? Why couldn't I just lie like my mother? Wasn't that easier?

- Where's your lunch?

- Um, I'm not hungry..

- Okay, have a seat Ashley.

- Mr. Anderson, why did you say my Grandparents should be worried?

- Ashley, you said you were being abused at home.

- But they aren't abusing me!

- I'm confused..

- Mr. Anderson, I had to move here with my Grandparents because I was taken away from my mother and Stepfather.

- Still listening..

- My stepfather was the one abusing me, and my Grandparents took me in.

- But you were crying over your Grandmother yesterday?

- Yeah, my Great Grandmother that died a few weeks ago.

- Don't you think we should go talk to the school counselor?

- Not yet please.

- Why?

- My mother forced me lie to the counselor and the principal about why I moved here so close to the end of the school year.

- I see, but you know we are not done talking about this.

- Okay, can I go now?

- Yes, and eat something. See you in class.

Oh boy, I still had to sit through class with him?

What have I done? Oh please how can I undo this?

Somehow I made it through two more classes, a run in

with him in the hallway and back to his room for business class or was it computer class? No matter he asked me to see him after class. Great he wants me to stay afterschool.

It seems like only 5 minutes have passed and I am back sitting in his classroom. You wouldn't think there would be much more to say at this point. I was suspicious and closed my mouth other then the begging him not to involve my Grandparents.

He started asking me questions; oh boy he was one of those. Already the gym teacher was asking me questions after hearing rumors I didn't eat lunch. He really only cared about my physical health anyway. Mr. Anderson actually seemed to care, pity that I couldn't let him in. Soon everything started going downhill.

I guess not terrible, I just couldn't concentrate. The gym teacher, Mr. Anderson, and even my government teacher took notice. No offense to Mr. Hoff, but really who could pay attention in Government?

Mr. Anderson kept talking to me, while my gym teacher was taking special notice in my weight. My Government teacher got in the mix too because he was concerned about my grades. Did I mention English was really my best subject?

Overtime I got more comfortable talking with Mr. Anderson, and hey it got me out of study halls. He wasn't just talking to me about stuff he was actually tutoring me and helping me get class work done. Joseph and he would have gotten along. There were only a few times Mr. Anderson got firm with me, but he was usually forgiving. I saw the times he had to get tough on students, I didn't want to be one of them.

He eventually did have me tell the school counselor the truth about why I had moved there. I resisted until he really gave me no choice. I still tried to get out of it but it was not too bad. After I confirmed that I was currently in safe situation, they backed off a bit.

Yeah, they backed down on that but kept an eye on my weight. I eventually managed to even get the gym teacher off my back for awhile. It happened in waves and Mr. Anderson kept looking after me.

Joseph and Mr. Anderson helped me muddle through those awkward years of high school. I was able to call Mr. Anderson a few years ago and thank him for what he did for me. I'm not sure if I can ever properly thank him, how can you repay someone that supported you at your worst?

I still wish I could find Joseph and thank him. If it wasn't for him I do not think I could have spoke up and allowed my friend to turn in my stepdad. After Joseph was terminated for helping me, I knew I had to do something. I wished I could have talked to him one last time, not even a chance to say goodbye.

Note from the Author:

Hello, I hope you enjoyed this introduction to my book the

Black Sheep. I am planning on writing more but I am

looking for feedback at this point. Thank you for reading.

www.ingramcontent.com/pod-product-compliance
Lightning Source LLC
Chambersburg PA
CBHW081733170526
45167CB00009B/3808